Beauty Beyond 40

BEAUTY TIPS FOR WOMEN 40 AND BEYOND

BY EMILY LAURA

EMILY LAURA

Beauty Beyond 40

Beautiful tips for women 40 and beyond

Copyright © 2023 by Emily Laura

All rights reserved. No part of this publication may be reproduced, stored or transmitted in any form or by any means, electronic, mechanical, photocopying, recording, scanning, or otherwise without written permission from the publisher. It is illegal to copy this book, post it to a website, or distribute it by any other means without permission.

Emily Laura asserts the moral right to be identified as the author of this work.

First edition

This book was professionally typeset on Reedsy. Find out more at reedsy.com

Contents

1	Introduction: Embracing the Timeless Beauty Within	1
2	Understanding Changes in Mature Skin	4
3	Enhancing Natural Beauty with Makeup	13
4	Nurturing Your Tresses: Haircare Advice for a Healthy and...	19
5	Nurturing Mind and Body: Fitness and Wellness check for...	32
6	Self-Care and Confidence Boosters	42
7	Embracing the Wisdom and Beauty of Aging	54
8	Conclusion	57

1

Introduction: Embracing the Timeless Beauty Within

Hello, Dear Friend,

I am absolutely thrilled to have you here, ready to embark on a journey that celebrates the breathtaking beauty that gracefully emerges as we enter the marvelous years of 40 and beyond. This is a guide crafted with love, designed specifically for extraordinary women like us, who understand that age is not a barrier to beauty, but a gateway to a whole new level of self-discovery and self-expression.

In a world that often idolizes youth and narrowly defines beauty, let us take a moment to redefine the standards and embrace the magnificence that comes with the passing of time. Together, we will delve into the captivating realm of self-care, where we will uncover skincare rituals that nurture and restore our radiant glow. We'll explore the wonders of makeup, discovering how to enhance our unique features and unleash our inner confidence.

And oh, the joy of haircare! We will celebrate the versatility of our locks, whether they're cascading waves, silver strands, or any other glorious form, as we unlock the secrets to embracing our individual beauty.

But, my dear, our journey is not only about the external. It is about the very essence of who we are—the wisdom, strength, and resilience that have shaped us into the remarkable women we have become. It is about nurturing our minds, bodies, and souls, with the understanding that true beauty radiates from within.

Let us embark on the path of wellness and self-discovery, exploring the invigorating power of exercise, mindful practices, and self-care rituals that replenish our spirits. We will celebrate the joy of movement, discovering activities that bring us immense pleasure and keep us feeling strong and vibrant. Together, we will unlock the transformative magic of embracing our authentic selves, igniting a fire within our souls that radiates an irresistible allure.

And, of course, we cannot forget the enchantment of fashion and style! Let us revel in the thrill of dressing for success, embracing our unique tastes, and celebrating the magnificent shapes of our bodies. From selecting the perfect outfit to finding the colors and patterns that make our hearts sing, we will tap into the art of sartorial expression, unleashing our inner fashionistas with confidence and flair.

Throughout this journey, my dear friend, remember that you are not alone. You are part of a community of extraordinary women,

INTRODUCTION: EMBRACING THE TIMELESS BEAUTY WITHIN

each with her own story, dreams, and aspirations. Together, we will uplift and support one another, celebrating the beauty that transcends age, societal norms, and expectations.

So, my dear, I invite you to join me on this incredible adventure of self-love, self-expression, and unapologetic authenticity. Together, let us revel in the undeniable beauty that resides within each and every one of us, illuminating the world with our unique radiance.

With all my heart,

[Emily Laura]

2

Understanding Changes in Mature Skin

One common change in mature skin is a decrease in elasticity. This means that our skin becomes less firm and more prone to wrinkles and sagging. To address this, look for skincare products that contain ingredients like peptides and retinol, which can help improve the firmness and resilience of your skin. Additionally, facial exercises and massage techniques can be beneficial in toning your facial muscles and promoting blood circulation.

Another concern is the loss of moisture and hydration. Mature skin tends to be drier, leading to dryness, flakiness, and a dull appearance. To combat this, prioritize hydration in your skincare routine by using moisturizers with hydrating ingredients like hyaluronic acid, ceramides, and natural oils. These ingredients help replenish and lock in moisture, giving your skin a refreshed and youthful glow.

Uneven skin tone and hyperpigmentation are also common in

mature skin. Sun damage and hormonal changes can cause dark spots and uneven pigmentation. Look for skincare products with brightening ingredients like vitamin C, niacinamide, or kojic acid to help fade these spots and even out your skin tone. Remember to protect your skin from further damage by wearing sunscreen daily.

Sensitive skin can become more prevalent as we age. It's important to choose gentle, fragrance-free products that nourish and soothe your skin. Look for skincare formulations designed for sensitive skin and consider using antioxidant-rich ingredients like green tea extract, chamomile, or aloe vera to calm and strengthen your skin's barrier.

Lastly, embrace self-care and self-acceptance on this journey. Aging is a natural part of life, and it should be celebrated. Take pride in the wisdom lines and other signs of aging on your face. Approach your skincare routine with love, patience, and gratitude for the unique beauty of your mature skin.

Nurturing Your Skin with Love and Care

Our skin, like a cherished companion, has accompanied us throughout life's adventures. It has witnessed our joys, our struggles, and everything in between. Through my own journey, I have come to understand the profound impact that nurturing our skin can have on our overall well-being. It is a deeply personal and self-empowering practice, and I am thrilled to guide you through it.

Let's start with the foundation of any effective **skincare routine:** cleansing. I have tried countless cleansers in my quest for a gentle yet effective formula. And let me tell you, finding the perfect match is like discovering a soulmate for your skin. I encourage you to explore various cleansers, paying attention to your skin's unique needs. For me, a soothing milk cleanser has worked wonders, delicately removing impurities while leaving my skin feeling supple and refreshed. As you cleanse your face, take a moment to savor the sensation, relishing in the simple act of self-care.

Ah!, **Exfoliation**—the secret to unveiling a radiant complexion. Through trial and error, I have learned the importance of exfoliating with intention and moderation. Over-enthusiastic exfoliation can disrupt the skin's delicate balance, so I now opt for a gentle exfoliator with natural ingredients, using it once or twice a week. The sensation of sloughing away dead skin cells is not only invigorating but also symbolic—a reminder that we can shed the old and embrace the new. As you exfoliate, visualize a fresh start, both for your skin and your spirit.

But skincare goes beyond mere external pampering; it is an opportunity for self-reflection and self-love. I have discovered the profound impact of incorporating self-care rituals into my skincare routine. For me, it's the act of applying a face mask that truly allows me to reconnect with myself. I choose masks infused with nourishing ingredients like honey or botanical extracts, reveling in the indulgent scent and texture. As I apply the mask, I take a few moments to unwind, allowing the cares of the day to melt away. It's a precious time to nurture not only my skin but also my soul.

As we navigate the realm of skincare, we must honor the changes that come with age. Through my own journey, I have learned to embrace the signs of wisdom that grace my face—the gentle lines that tell stories of laughter, resilience, and growth. I now seek out products that cater specifically to mature skin, with ingredients like hyaluronic acid and antioxidants. These formulations have helped restore elasticity and radiance, reminding me that beauty is not confined to youth but is a tapestry woven with the threads of experience.

Remember, dear friend, skincare is not a superficial pursuit but a daily ritual of self-love. As we follow the steps and recommendations in this chapter, I invite you to infuse them with your own personal touch. Let your skincare routine become a sanctuary a space for reflection, self-acceptance, and celebration of the remarkable canvas that is your skin.

Cleansing and Moisturizing Tips for Mature Skin

Cleansing Tips:

1. **Choose a gentle cleanser:** Opt for a cleanser specifically formulated for mature skin. Look for mild, non-drying cleansers that contain ingredients like hyaluronic acid or ceramides. These ingredients help retain moisture and protect the skin's natural barrier. Avoid harsh cleansers that can strip away essential oils and leave your skin feeling dry.

2. **Use lukewarm water:** When cleansing your face, use lukewarm water instead of hot water. Hot water can be drying and irritating to mature skin. Using lukewarm water helps maintain a healthy moisture balance and prevents excessive dryness.

3. **Be gentle:** Treat your skin with care by using gentle, circular motions when cleansing. Avoid harsh scrubbing or pulling on the skin, as this can lead to irritation and increased sensitivity. Pat your skin dry with a soft towel instead of rubbing it vigorously.

4. **Double cleansing:** Consider using the double cleansing method, especially if you wear makeup or sunscreen. Start with an oil-based cleanser to dissolve and remove impurities, followed by a water-based cleanser to thoroughly cleanse your skin. This method ensures a deep cleanse and removes all traces of makeup and dirt.

Moisturizing Tips:

1. **Hydrate your skin:** Moisturizing is essential for mature skin as it helps replenish lost moisture and maintain a plump and supple complexion. Look for moisturizers with hydrating ingredients like hyaluronic acid, glycerin, or ceramides. These ingredients attract and retain moisture in the skin, keeping it hydrated throughout the day.

2. **Don't forget the neck and decolletage:** Extend your moisturizing routine beyond your face and apply moisturizer to

your neck and décolletage as well. These areas are prone to showing signs of aging and benefit from regular hydration. Gently massage the moisturizer into these areas using upward motions.

3. **Consider a heavier moisturizer for nighttime:** Nighttime is an opportunity for your skin to repair and regenerate. Consider using a slightly heavier moisturizer or incorporating a hydrating overnight mask to provide intense hydration and nourishment while you sleep. This allows your skin to wake up refreshed and rejuvenated.

4. **Protect with sunscreen:** Sun protection is crucial for maintaining the health and appearance of mature skin. Use a broad-spectrum sunscreen with SPF 30 or higher daily, even on cloudy days or when indoors. Apply it generously to your face, neck, and any exposed areas to shield your skin from harmful UV rays and prevent further damage.

Remember to listen to your skin and adjust your cleansing and moisturizing routine as needed. Everyone's skin is unique, so pay attention to how your skin reacts to different products and make changes accordingly.

Embracing the Power of Serums and Face Oils

In our journey to nurture and revitalize our mature skin, we often seek out anti-aging products that promise to unlock the fountain of youth. Today, we'll dive into the captivating world of serums and face oils two extraordinary allies that can work wonders for our skin as we age.

Let's start with serums, those little magical potions that pack a punch of powerful ingredients. They are like concentrated elixirs, meticulously formulated to penetrate deeply into the skin and deliver potent nourishment where it's needed most. What makes serums truly remarkable is their lightweight texture, which allows for easy absorption and swift results. They're like secret weapons in our skincare arsenal, targeting specific concerns like fine lines, wrinkles, uneven skin tone, and loss of firmness.

When it comes to choosing the right serum for our skin, it's essential to look beyond the fancy marketing claims and focus on the ingredients that truly make a difference. Let's explore some of these remarkable ingredients that have stood the test of time:

1. **Retinol**: Ah, the superhero of anti-aging! Retinol, derived from vitamin A, is renowned for its remarkable ability to stimulate collagen production, improve skin texture, and reduce the appearance of fine lines and wrinkles. It's like a time-traveling ingredient that brings back the youthful glow we once possessed. When using retinol, it's important to start with a low concentration and gradually increase as our skin becomes more accustomed to its effects.

2. **Vitamin C:** The radiant beauty of vitamin C is hard to ignore. This powerful antioxidant not only brightens our skin but also

helps fade dark spots and promotes collagen synthesis. It's like a burst of sunshine for our faces, illuminating and rejuvenating our complexion. Seek out serums enriched with vitamin C for that extra dose of luminosity.

3. **Hyaluronic Acid:** When it comes to hydration, hyaluronic acid is a true hero. This natural molecule has an incredible ability to attract and retain moisture, plumping up our skin and restoring its youthful resilience. Think of it as a drink of water for our skin, quenching its thirst and revealing a dewy and supple complexion.

Now, let's shift our attention to the enchanting world of face oils. These luxurious elixirs have been cherished for centuries for their ability to nourish and replenish the skin. Face oils are like precious potions, derived from various botanical extracts, rich in antioxidants, fatty acids, and vitamins. They provide deep hydration, strengthen the skin barrier, and restore a radiant glow.

Incorporating face oils into our skincare routine can be a transformative experience. They provide an extra layer of protection, sealing in moisture and shielding our skin from environmental stressors. Face oils effortlessly glide onto our skin, indulging our senses and allowing us to create a tranquil moment of self-care. The key is to choose oils that are suitable for our skin type—whether it's lightweight oils like jojoba and rosehip for oily or combination skin, or richer oils like argan and avocado for dry or mature skin.

As we embrace serums and face oils, let us remember that

skincare is not just a series of steps; it's a beautiful ritual of self-love and self-discovery. The application of serums and face oils becomes a moment of connection with ourselves, as we gently massage these exquisite elixirs into our skin, nurturing it with tenderness and care.

3

Enhancing Natural Beauty with Makeup

Makeup is a powerful tool that allows us to express ourselves and enhance our natural beauty. In this chapter, we will explore the art of enhancing our features through makeup, embracing our unique qualities and radiating confidence. Whether you're a makeup aficionado or new to the world of cosmetics, these tips will help you enhance your natural beauty in a way that feels authentic and empowering.

1. Start with Skincare:

Before diving into makeup, it's essential to prioritize skincare. Cleanse and moisturize your skin daily to create a healthy canvas. Remember, well-nourished and hydrated skin is the foundation for a flawless makeup application.

2. Embrace the Power of a Subtle Base:

When it comes to foundation, less is often more. Aim for a lightweight formula that allows your skin to breathe while providing subtle coverage. Choose a shade that matches your skin tone to create a seamless and natural look. Apply the foundation sparingly, focusing on areas that need a bit of evening out, and blend it gently using a sponge or brush.

3. Accentuate Your Eyes:

The eyes are the windows to the soul, so let's make them shine! Start by grooming your eyebrows to frame your face beautifully. Fill in any sparse areas with a brow pencil or powder for a defined yet natural appearance. Next, apply eyeshadow shades that enhance your eye color and complement your skin tone. Soft, neutral tones work well for everyday looks, while deeper hues can add depth and drama for special occasions.

4. Enhance Your Lashes:

Luscious lashes can instantly elevate your look. Curl your lashes using an eyelash curler and apply mascara to add volume and length. If desired, you can also opt for false lashes for a more dramatic effect. Remember to choose a mascara that is suitable for your lash type and always apply it with a light hand to avoid clumping.

5. Create a Radiant Complexion:

A healthy glow can make you look vibrant and youthful. Add a touch of blush to the apples of your cheeks for a natural flush of color. Opt for shades that complement your skin tone and blend it softly for a seamless finish. Additionally, use a subtle highlighter to enhance your cheekbones, brow bone, and cupid's bow. This will give your face a luminous and radiant appearance.

6. Emphasize Your Lips:

Your lips are a beautiful canvas for self-expression. Choose lip colors that flatter your skin tone and match the mood you want to convey. From soft pinks to bold reds, experiment with different shades to find what makes you feel confident and empowered. Don't forget to prep your lips with a moisturizing balm to keep them smooth and hydrated throughout the day.

7. **Set Your Makeup:**
To make your makeup last longer, use a setting spray or powder to lock it in place. This step will help control shine and ensure your hard work stays intact throughout the day or evening.

Makeup is not about masking your features but enhancing the beauty that already exists within you. By following these tips, you can create a makeup look that accentuates your natural attributes, boosts your self-confidence, and reflects your unique personality. Remember, makeup is an art form, and it's all about finding what makes you feel beautiful and comfortable in your own skin.

Mastering Long-Lasting Makeup: Tips for a Flawless Look

There's nothing more frustrating than spending time perfecting your makeup only to have it fade away or smudge throughout the day. In this chapter, we'll delve into the secrets of long-lasting makeup, so you can enjoy a flawless look that withstands the test of time. Whether you have a busy day ahead or a special occasion to attend, these tips will help your makeup stay put and keep you looking fabulous.

1. **Prep Your Skin:**

Prepping your skin is crucial for long-lasting makeup. Start by cleansing your face to remove any excess oil or dirt. Follow up with a lightweight moisturizer that suits your skin type. Hydrated skin creates a smooth canvas for makeup application and helps it adhere better.

2. **Use a Primer:**

Primer acts as a base for your makeup, creating a smooth and even surface. Choose a primer that suits your skin concerns, such as mattifying for oily skin or illuminating for a radiant glow. Apply a small amount of primer all over your face, focusing on areas where your makeup tends to fade, such as the T-zone or around the nose.

3. **Choose Long-Wearing Products:**

Opt for long-wearing and waterproof formulas when selecting your makeup products. Look for keywords like "long-lasting," "transfer-resistant," or "smudge-proof" on product labels. These formulations are designed to stay put and resist fading, smudging, or melting throughout the day.

4. **Set Your Foundation:**

To ensure your foundation lasts, set it with a light dusting of translucent powder. This step helps absorb excess oil and prevents your foundation from sliding off your face. Use a fluffy brush to gently sweep the powder over your T-zone and other areas prone to shine.

5. Invest in Quality Brushes and Tools:

Using the right brushes and tools can make a significant difference in how your makeup wears and blends. Invest in high-quality brushes that are soft, durable, and designed for specific purposes. Good brushes help distribute products evenly and ensure a seamless application, contributing to the longevity of your makeup.

6. Layer and Build:

When applying eyeshadow or blush, layering and building the color gradually can make it more long-lasting. Start with a light application and gradually intensify the color as needed. This technique helps the pigments adhere better to your skin and prevents them from fading throughout the day.

7. Set Your Makeup with Setting Spray:

After completing your makeup, finish it off with a setting spray. Setting sprays create a fine mist that helps lock your makeup in place. They not only extend the wear of your makeup but also provide a fresh and hydrated look. Hold the bottle about an arm's length away from your face and spritz a few times for an even distribution.

8. Carry Essentials for Touch-Ups:

Even with the best long-lasting makeup, touch-ups may be necessary, especially in areas prone to oiliness or smudging. Carry a small makeup bag with a compact powder, blotting papers, a lip color, and a small brush for any quick fixes throughout the day.

With these tips for long-lasting makeup, you can confidently rock your flawless look from morning till night. Proper skincare, the right products, and a few strategic steps ensure that your makeup remains fresh, vibrant, and intact. Don't let the fear of makeup meltdown hold you back—embrace the day with confidence, knowing that your makeup is here to stay.

4

Nurturing Your Tresses: Haircare Advice for a Healthy and Beautiful Mane

Our hair is a reflection of our identity and plays a significant role in how we feel about ourselves. As we age, our hair may undergo changes in texture, thickness, and color. Let's embrace our unique hair journey and discover how to nurture our tresses with love and care.

1. Understand Your Hair Type:

Every individual has a unique hair type, whether it's straight, wavy, curly, or coily. Understanding your hair type is crucial in determining the right products and techniques for its care. Take some time to observe and appreciate your hair's natural texture, as this will guide you in choosing the most suitable products and hairstyles.

2. **Gentle Cleansing:**

When it comes to washing your hair, opt for a gentle shampoo that doesn't strip away natural oils. Avoid harsh sulfates and look for nourishing ingredients that promote hydration and moisture. Massage the shampoo into your scalp using your fingertips, stimulating blood circulation and ensuring a thorough cleanse.

3. **Condition for Softness and Hydration:**
Conditioning is key to maintaining soft, manageable, and hydrated hair. After shampooing, apply a conditioner from mid-length to the ends, focusing on the areas that tend to be drier. Leave the conditioner on for a few minutes before rinsing it out. This step helps replenish moisture, detangle knots, and improve overall hair health.

4. **Embrace Deep Conditioning Treatments:**
Treat your hair to a deep conditioning treatment once or twice a month to restore moisture, repair damage, and promote hair strength. Look for masks or treatments specifically formulated for your hair type or concerns. Apply the treatment generously, focusing on the lengths and ends, and leave it on for the recommended time for maximum benefits.

5. **Protect Your Hair from Heat:**
Excessive heat styling can damage your hair over time, leading to dryness and breakage. Minimize the use of heat tools such as blow dryers, flat irons, and curling irons. When you do use them, apply a heat protectant spray or serum to shield your hair from the high temperatures. Opt for air-drying or try heatless styling techniques whenever possible.

6. **Be Mindful of Hair Color:**
If you choose to color your hair, be mindful of the products

and techniques used. Harsh chemicals can weaken and damage the hair shaft, making it more susceptible to breakage. Consider opting for ammonia-free or semi-permanent hair dyes, and always follow up with a deep conditioning treatment to maintain the health and vibrancy of your color-treated locks.

7. Trim Regularly:

Regular trims are essential for keeping your hair healthy and free from split ends. Aim for a trim every 8 to 12 weeks, depending on your hair's growth rate. Trimming removes damaged ends, promotes hair growth, and keeps your mane looking fresh and vibrant.

8. **Nourish from Within:**

Remember, healthy hair starts from within. Maintain a balanced diet, rich in nutrients such as vitamins A, C, E, biotin, and omega-3 fatty acids. Stay hydrated by drinking plenty of water to keep your hair moisturized and promote overall hair health.

Your hair is a unique and beautiful part of who you are. By embracing your hair's natural texture, using gentle cleansing and conditioning techniques, protecting it from heat, and nourishing it from within, you can maintain a healthy and beautiful mane. Let your hair be an expression of your individuality and embrace the joy of caring for it with love and appreciation.

Embracing Change: Dealing with Thinning Hair and Hair Loss

Hair loss and thinning hair can be a sensitive and challenging experience, impacting our self-esteem and confidence. It's essential to recognize that you are not alone in this journey and that there are practical steps you can take to address these concerns. In this chapter, we'll explore the causes of thinning hair and hair loss, as well as delve into comprehensive strategies to help you embrace the changes and feel empowered in your own skin.

1. **Understand the Causes:**

Thinning hair and hair loss can have various underlying causes, including hormonal changes, genetics, stress, nutritional deficiencies, certain medications, and medical conditions such as alopecia. It's important to consult with a healthcare professional or a dermatologist to determine the specific cause of your hair loss. Understanding the root cause can guide you towards appropriate solutions and treatments.

2. **Nourish Your Hair:**

Taking care of your hair from the inside out is crucial for promoting its health and growth. Ensure you have a well-balanced diet that includes essential nutrients like protein, biotin, vitamins A, C, and E, and omega-3 fatty acids. Consider incorporating hair supplements recommended by your healthcare professional to support hair health. Additionally, choose haircare products that are gentle, nourishing, and free from harsh chemicals. Look for shampoos, conditioners, and treatments specifically formulated for thinning hair or hair loss, which often contain ingredients like biotin, keratin, collagen, and essential oils to nourish the scalp and strengthen the hair follicles.

3. **Gentle Hair Handling:**

When dealing with thinning hair, it's crucial to handle it with care to prevent further breakage and damage. Avoid aggressive brushing or combing, as this can lead to hair fall. Opt for a wide-toothed comb or a brush with soft bristles to gently detangle your hair, starting from the ends and working your way up. Be mindful of tight hairstyles or excessive pulling, which can put unnecessary stress on the hair follicles. Consider using hair-friendly accessories like silk scrunchies or gentle hair ties to minimize breakage.

4. **Volumizing Techniques:**

Experiment with different styling techniques to create the illusion of volume and thickness. Use volumizing mousses, sprays, or dry shampoos to add texture and lift to your roots. Consider blow-drying your hair upside down to create more volume at the roots. Incorporate gentle teasing or backcombing techniques to add fullness to specific areas. Hairstyles such as loose curls, waves, or updos with strategically placed pins or accessories can also give the appearance of fuller hair.

5. **Consult a Hairstylist:**

Seek guidance from a professional hairstylist who specializes in working with thinning hair. They can provide valuable insights and suggest suitable haircuts, styles, and products to enhance the appearance of volume and thickness. A skilled hairstylist can also teach you techniques to camouflage thinning areas, create strategic layering, or incorporate extensions or hairpieces to add fullness. Regular visits to your hairstylist for trims can help maintain the health and shape of your hair.

6. Consider Hair Extensions or Wigs:

Hair extensions or wigs can be temporary solutions to add volume and length to your hair while you work on improving its health. Consult with a reputable hair extension specialist or wig provider to find the most suitable option for you. High-quality extensions or wigs can look natural and boost your confidence. Ensure that you properly care for and maintain them to prevent any damage to your existing hair.

7. **Explore Medical Treatments:**

In cases where hair loss is caused by underlying medical conditions, there are various medical treatments available. Topical minoxidil, approved by

the FDA for hair regrowth, can be effective in slowing down hair loss and stimulating regrowth. Other prescription medications, such as finasteride, may be recommended for specific types of hair loss. These treatments should be discussed and prescribed by a medical professional who can evaluate your specific situation and provide appropriate guidance.

8. **Embrace Your Natural Beauty:**

While dealing with thinning hair and hair loss can be challenging, it's important to embrace your natural beauty and focus on self-acceptance. Experiment with different hairstyles, accessories, or makeup techniques that highlight your best features and make you feel confident and beautiful. Emphasize your eyes, play with vibrant lip colors, or focus on flawless skin to enhance your overall appearance. Remember that your worth extends far beyond your hair, and cultivating self-love and self-acceptance is the key to radiating beauty.

Dealing with thinning hair and hair loss requires patience, self-care, and a proactive approach. By understanding the causes, nourishing your hair, seeking professional guidance, considering styling techniques, and exploring available treatments, you can navigate this journey with grace and confidence. Embrace your unique beauty, celebrate your inner strength, and remember that your beauty shines from within, regardless of any physical changes.

Embracing the Spectrum: Color and Highlights for Mature Hair

Hair color has the power to transform our look and boost our confidence. As we age, our hair may naturally lose pigment, and grays or whites may appear. In this chapter, we'll explore the exciting world of hair color and highlights for mature hair. Whether you want to enhance your natural shade, cover grays, or experiment with a new look, we'll provide detailed guidance and explanation to help you embrace the spectrum and find a color that makes you feel fabulous.

1. **Consult with a Professional Colorist:**

When it comes to coloring mature hair, it's essential to consult with a professional colorist who has experience working with different hair types and textures. A skilled colorist can assess your hair's condition, discuss your desired outcome, and recommend suitable colors and techniques that complement your skin tone and enhance your features. They can also advise on the best approach to cover grays or achieve a natural-looking result.

2. **Enhancing Your Natural Shade:**

If you want to enhance your natural hair color, consider opting for a shade that complements your skin tone and blends seamlessly with your existing color. For a subtle and natural-looking change, choose a color that is one to two shades lighter or darker than your natural hue. This can help add depth, dimension, and shine to your hair while maintaining a cohesive look.

3. **Covering Grays:**

Many women choose to color their hair to cover grays and regain a more youthful appearance. If you're aiming to cover grays, it's important to discuss this with your colorist. They can recommend hair dye formulations that provide optimal gray coverage while still delivering a natural-looking result. Consider shades close to your natural color or choose a color that matches your desired look.

4. **Highlights and Lowlights:**

Highlights and lowlights can add depth, dimension, and texture to mature hair, creating a vibrant and youthful appearance.

Opt for subtle highlights or lowlights that complement your base color and skin tone. Soft, multidimensional shades like caramel, honey, or golden tones can beautifully blend with your natural hair color and create a sun-kissed effect. Balayage and foil techniques are commonly used for a seamless and natural look.

5. **Balancing Warmth and Cool Tones:**

As we age, our skin tone may change, and it's important to consider this when choosing hair colors. Warm tones like golden blondes, rich browns, or copper shades can add warmth to the complexion and impart a radiant glow. Cool tones like ash blondes, cool browns, or platinum shades can create a sophisticated and chic look. Work with your colorist to find the right balance of warm and cool tones that flatter your skin tone and bring out your best features.

6. **Maintenance and Care:**

Colored hair requires proper maintenance and care to keep it looking vibrant and healthy. Use color-safe shampoos and conditioners formulated specifically for color-treated hair to prevent color fading and maintain moisture balance. Deep conditioning treatments can help nourish and restore the hair's health. Protect your hair from excessive sun exposure by wearing hats or using UV protection sprays. Regular touch-ups and trims can help maintain the desired color and keep your hair looking fresh and lively.

7. **Embrace Change and Experiment:**

Hair color is a fantastic opportunity to express your creativity and embrace change. Don't be afraid to step out of your comfort zone and try something new. If you've always been a brunette, consider exploring shades of red or blonde. Play with highlights, lowlights, or even trendy techniques like ombre or balayage. Remember that hair color is a temporary change, so don't be afraid to experiment and have fun with it.

Coloring your hair is an exciting way to express your personal style and enhance your natural beauty. With the guidance of a professional colorist, you can achieve a stunning and natural-looking result that boosts your confidence and makes you feel fabulous. Embrace the spectrum of hair colors, whether you want to enhance your natural shade, cover grays, or experiment with highlights and lowlights. Maintain your colored hair with proper care and enjoy the transformative power of hair color as you embrace change and embrace your unique beauty.

Caring for Gray Hair

Gray hair is a beautiful and natural part of the aging process, symbolizing wisdom and grace. In this chapter, we'll delve into the essential tips and techniques for caring for gray hair, ensuring that it looks radiant, healthy, and full of life. Whether you're embracing your natural silver strands or considering transitioning to gray, we'll provide you with valuable insights on how to care for and maintain your gorgeous gray locks.

1. Embrace the Transition:
If you're in the process of transitioning to gray hair, it's important to embrace the journey. Patience is key as your hair

grows out and the natural gray color becomes more prominent. Avoid using harsh chemical dyes or bleaches to cover your gray, as they can damage your hair and hinder the transition process. Instead, work with your hairstylist to develop a gradual transition plan that allows your gray hair to blend seamlessly with your existing color.

2. Optimal Shampoo and Conditioner:

Gray hair has unique characteristics that require specific care. Look for shampoos and conditioners formulated for gray or silver hair. These products help enhance the brightness of your gray strands, reduce yellowing or brassiness, and provide moisture to keep your hair soft and manageable. Avoid using products that contain sulfates, as they can strip the hair of its natural oils, making it dry and brittle.

3. Regular Deep Conditioning:

Gray hair tends to be more susceptible to dryness and frizz. To combat these issues, incorporate regular deep conditioning treatments into your hair care routine. Choose deep conditioning masks or treatments that are hydrating and nourishing. Apply the product to your hair, focusing on the mid-lengths and ends, and leave it on for the recommended time. This will help restore moisture, improve hair elasticity, and leave your gray hair looking smooth and lustrous.

4. Combating Yellowing:

One common concern with gray hair is yellowing or dullness. This can be caused by various factors, such as environmental pollutants or product buildup. To combat yellowing, use a purple or blue toning shampoo once or twice a month. These shampoos help neutralize the yellow tones in your hair, keeping it bright and vibrant. Be cautious not to overuse toning shampoos, as they can leave a bluish or purple cast if used excessively.

5. **Protect from UV Damage:**

Gray hair is more prone to sun damage, as it lacks the natural pigment that provides protection. To shield your gray locks from harmful UV rays, use hair products that contain UV filters or wear a hat when spending extended periods in the sun. Additionally, consider using leave-in conditioners or serums with UV protection to keep your hair hydrated and shielded from damage.

6. **Minimize Heat Styling:**

Excessive heat styling can cause dryness and breakage, which is especially noticeable on gray hair. Minimize the use of heat styling tools like blow dryers, curling irons, and straighteners. When you do style your hair with heat, use a heat protectant spray to create a barrier and reduce the risk of damage. Embrace air-drying or opt for heatless styling techniques to maintain the health and integrity of your gray strands.

7. **Regular Trims:**

Regular trims are essential for maintaining healthy and vibrant-looking gray hair. Trimming your hair every six to eight weeks helps remove split ends and prevents them from traveling up the hair shaft. This not only improves the overall appearance of your hair but also promotes healthier growth.

8. **Embrace Texture and Hairstyles:**

Gray hair often has a unique texture and can be coarser or more wiry compared to pigmented hair. Embrace and celebrate this texture by choosing hairstyles that complement your natural gray hair. Consult with a hairstylist who has experience working with gray hair and can recommend styles that enhance your features and suit your hair type. Consider embracing your natural waves, curls, or opting for shorter styles that require less maintenance.

Caring for gray hair is all about embracing its natural beauty and providing it with the specific care it needs. By following these tips, you can keep your gray hair radiant, healthy, and full of life. Embrace the transition process, choose suitable hair care products, and protect your gray strands from yellowing and UV damage. With proper care and attention, your gray hair will shine and serve as a testament to your beauty, wisdom, and self-confidence.

5

Nurturing Mind and Body: Fitness and Wellness check for Longevity

Maintaining a healthy and active lifestyle is crucial for long-term wellness and vitality.

1. **Holistic Approach to Fitness:**

As we age, it's important to adopt a holistic approach to fitness that encompasses cardiovascular exercise, strength training, flexibility, and balance exercises. Engaging in a variety of activities helps promote overall physical fitness, improve cardiovascular health, build muscle strength, enhance flexibility, and reduce the risk of falls and injuries. Consult with a fitness professional or personal trainer to develop a personalized exercise plan tailored to your needs and abilities.

2. **Cardiovascular Exercise:**

Regular cardiovascular exercise is essential for maintaining heart health, boosting energy levels, and managing weight. Engage in activities such as brisk walking, swimming, cycling, or dancing to get your heart rate up and increase endurance. Aim for at least 150 minutes of moderate-intensity aerobic exercise or 75 minutes of vigorous-intensity exercise per week, as recommended by health authorities.

3. **Strength Training:**

Strength training helps preserve muscle mass, increase bone density, and improve overall strength and functional abilities. Incorporate resistance exercises using weights, resistance bands, or bodyweight exercises into your routine. Focus on all major muscle groups, including arms, legs, core, and back. Start with lighter weights and gradually increase as you build strength and confidence. Aim for strength training exercises two to three times per week.

4. **Flexibility and Balance:**

Flexibility and balance exercises are essential for maintaining joint mobility, preventing injuries, and reducing the risk of falls. Include stretching exercises, yoga, tai chi, or Pilates in your fitness regimen to improve flexibility, posture, and balance. These activities also promote relaxation, reduce stress, and enhance overall well-being.

5. **Mindful Movement:**

Incorporate mindful movement practices such as yoga or meditation into your fitness routine. These practices not only improve physical flexibility and strength but also cultivate mental clarity, reduce stress, and promote a sense of calm and inner peace. Find a class or follow online tutorials that cater to your fitness level and preferences.

6. Nutrition and Hydration:

Support your fitness and wellness journey by nourishing your body with a balanced and nutritious diet. Consume a variety of whole foods, including fruits, vegetables, lean proteins, whole grains, and healthy fats. Stay hydrated by drinking an adequate amount of water throughout the day. Consult with a nutritionist or dietitian for personalized guidance based on your specific dietary needs and goals.

7. **Rest and Recovery:**

Rest and recovery are integral parts of any fitness and wellness routine. Allow your body to rest and regenerate by ensuring you get enough quality sleep each night. Listen to your body's cues and take rest days as needed to prevent overexertion and injury. Incorporate relaxation techniques such as deep breathing, meditation, or gentle stretching to promote restful sleep and overall well-being.

8. **Social Connections and Mental Well-being:**

Nurturing your mental well-being is just as important as physical fitness. Stay socially engaged by maintaining connections with friends, family, and community. Engage in activities that bring you joy and fulfillment, whether it's pursuing hobbies, volunteering, or joining social groups. Seek support from loved ones or consider professional help if you experience challenges in your mental well-being.

Fitness and wellness are lifelong journeys that require dedication, consistency, and a holistic approach. By prioritizing physical activity, nourishing your body with healthy foods, fostering mental well-being, and maintaining social connections, you can embrace a fulfilling and vibrant life.

Remember to listen to your body, adapt your fitness routine as needed, and celebrate the progress you make along the way. By nurturing your mind and body, you can cultivate a sense of well-being and enjoy the benefits of a healthy and active lifestyle for years to come.

Strategies for Stress Reduction and Inner Balance

In our modern, fast-paced world, stress has become a prevalent and often overwhelming aspect of our lives. However, effectively managing stress is crucial for maintaining our well-being and achieving inner balance. we will explore a range of proven strategies for stress reduction that can help you find equilibrium, enhance your mental and emotional health, and navigate life's challenges with resilience. By incorporating these techniques into your daily routine, you can cultivate a calmer, more centered mindset and experience greater overall well-being.

1. **Deep Breathing Techniques:**

Deep breathing exercises serve as powerful tools for stress reduction. By practicing controlled, deep breaths, you can activate your body's relaxation response and promote a sense of calm. Try diaphragmatic breathing, where you inhale deeply through your nose, allowing your abdomen to rise, and then exhale slowly through your mouth, allowing your abdomen to fall. This simple technique can be practiced anywhere and anytime stress arises.

2. **Mindfulness and Meditation:**

Mindfulness and meditation practices cultivate present-moment awareness and help quiet the mind. Through consistent practice, you can train your mind to observe thoughts and emotions without judgment. Set aside dedicated time each day for meditation, focusing on your breath, bodily sensations, or a specific point of focus. Over time, mindfulness and meditation can reduce stress, enhance clarity, and improve overall well-being.

3. **Regular Exercise:**

Physical activity is a potent stress reducer and mood enhancer. Engaging in regular exercise, whether it's cardiovascular workouts, strength training, yoga, or other forms of movement, releases endorphins and reduces stress hormones. Find activities that you enjoy and make them a consistent part of your routine. Aim for at least 30 minutes of moderate-intensity exercise most days of the week.

4. **Nature and Outdoor Exposure:**

Spending time in nature and immersing yourself in natural surroundings can have a profound impact on stress reduction. Take walks in parks, forests, or along the beach to reconnect with the calming rhythms of the natural world. The beauty and tranquility of nature provide a welcome respite from the demands of daily life, allowing for relaxation and rejuvenation.

5. **Cultivating Social Connections:**

Nurturing meaningful social connections is vital for managing stress and promoting well-being. Seek support from family, friends, or support groups during challenging times. Engage in regular social activities, such as shared hobbies, outings, or simply spending quality time together. Meaningful connections provide a sense of belonging, understanding, and support, which can significantly reduce stress levels.

6. **Effective Time Management:**

Managing time efficiently and setting realistic priorities are essential for stress reduction. Learn to identify your most important tasks and allocate your time accordingly. Break down larger projects into smaller, manageable steps, and set realistic deadlines. By organizing your time effectively, you can reduce stress levels and increase productivity, leaving room for relaxation and self-care.

7. **Engaging in Relaxation Techniques:**

Explore various relaxation techniques to find what works best for you. This may include practices such as progressive muscle relaxation, guided imagery, aromatherapy, or listening to calming music. Experiment with different techniques and incorporate them into your daily routine to promote relaxation, reduce tension, and alleviate stress.

8. **Self-Care and Personal Well-being:**

Prioritizing self-care is fundamental to managing stress effectively. Establish regular self-care practices that nurture your physical, mental, and emotional well-being. This may involve engaging in activities you enjoy, such as reading, taking baths, pursuing hobbies, practicing mindfulness, or engaging in creative outlets. Taking time for yourself replenishes your energy, enhances resilience, and promotes a healthier, more balanced life.

Implementing strategies for stress reduction is a lifelong journey that requires commitment and practice.

By incorporating deep breathing techniques, mindfulness and meditation, regular exercise, time in nature, nurturing social connections, effective time management, relaxation techniques, and prioritizing self-care, you can significantly reduce stress levels and cultivate inner balance. Remember, stress is a natural part of life, but with the right tools and mindset, you can navigate it with resilience and live a more fulfilling and harmonious life.

Nourishing Your Body: Nutrition Tips for Healthy Aging

As we age, maintaining a healthy and balanced diet becomes increasingly important for overall well-being and healthy aging. Proper nutrition provides essential nutrients, supports energy levels, strengthens the immune system, and reduces the risk of chronic diseases.

1. Eat a Varied and Colorful Diet:

Focus on consuming a wide variety of whole foods to ensure you receive a range of essential nutrients. Include plenty of colorful fruits and vegetables in your meals, as they are rich in vitamins, minerals, antioxidants, and fiber. Aim for a rainbow of colors on your plate to maximize nutrient intake and promote overall health.

2. Prioritize Nutrient-Dense Foods:

Choose nutrient-dense foods that provide a high concentration of vitamins, minerals, and other beneficial compounds per calorie. Incorporate lean proteins such as fish, poultry, legumes, and tofu into your diet. Opt for whole grains like quinoa, brown rice, and whole wheat bread. Include healthy fats from sources like avocados, nuts, seeds, and olive oil. These foods provide essential nutrients while keeping calorie intake in check.

3. Self-care Hydrated

Proper hydration is vital for maintaining overall health and well-being. Drink an adequate amount of water throughout the day to support digestion, circulation, and organ function. Keep a water bottle handy and sip water regularly, even if you don't feel thirsty. Limit the consumption of sugary beverages and opt for water, herbal tea, or infused water for hydration.

4. Mindful Eating:

Practice mindful eating to enhance your relationship with food and promote better digestion. Slow down and savor each bite, paying attention to your body's hunger and fullness cues. Avoid distractions like TV or screens while eating, allowing yourself to fully enjoy and appreciate the flavors and textures of your food. This practice can help prevent overeating and improve digestion.

5. Watch Portion Sizes:

As we age, our metabolism may slow down, and our calorie needs may decrease. Be mindful of portion sizes to avoid excessive calorie intake. Use smaller plates and bowls to help control portion sizes visually. Listen to your body's signals of hunger and fullness, stopping eating when you feel satisfied rather than overly full.

6. Adequate Protein Intake:

Maintain an adequate protein intake to support muscle strength and overall health. Include lean sources of protein such as lean meats, poultry, fish, eggs, dairy products, legumes, and plant-based protein sources like tofu and tempeh. Protein is essential for maintaining muscle mass, supporting immune function, and promoting healthy aging.

7. Mind the Micronutrients:

As we age, certain nutrients become especially important for maintaining optimal health. Ensure you're getting enough calcium and vitamin D to support bone health. Incorporate sources of vitamin B12, found in animal products or fortified foods, to support nerve function. Consider adding omega-3 fatty acids from fatty fish, flaxseeds, chia seeds, or walnuts to support heart and brain health.

8. Consult a Registered Dietitian:

If you have specific dietary concerns, health conditions, or need personalized guidance, consider consulting a registered dietitian. They can provide individualized recommendations based on your unique needs, help address nutritional deficiencies, and support you in making healthy choices that promote healthy aging.

Proper nutrition plays a crucial role in healthy aging and overall well-being. By following these nutrition tips, you can nourish your body, support optimal health, and enhance your quality of life as you age. Remember, small, sustainable changes in your eating habits can have a significant impact on your long term health and vitality.

6

Self-Care and Confidence Boosters

Self-care and building self-confidence have played transformative roles in my own life, and I'm excited to share their importance with you. Taking care of ourselves and nurturing our self-confidence are not selfish acts but essential for our overall well-being and happiness. By incorporating self-care practices and boosting our confidence, we can experience increased resilience, inner strength, and a greater sense of fulfillment.

1. Prioritizing Self-Care:

I've learned firsthand the power of prioritizing self-care. Making time for activities that bring me joy and relaxation, such as going for a walk in nature, reading a good book, or indulging in a pampering skincare routine, has had a profound impact on my mental and emotional well-being. By consciously dedicating time to self-care, we replenish our energy, reduce stress, and cultivate a positive mindset.

2. **Cultivating Positive Self-Talk:**
Throughout my journey, I've realized the tremendous influence our inner dialogue has on our self-confidence. Shifting from negative self-talk to positive affirmations and self-encouragement has been a game-changer for me. I remind myself of my strengths, celebrate my accomplishments, and practice self-compassion. By nurturing a positive internal dialogue, we can uplift our self-confidence and embrace our unique qualities.

3. **Setting Boundaries**:
Learning to set healthy boundaries has been a transformative aspect of my self-care journey. It was challenging at first, but I've discovered that establishing boundaries is crucial for maintaining my well-being and fostering self-respect. By communicating my needs and saying "no" when necessary, I've reclaimed control over my time and energy, allowing me to focus on activities and relationships that truly align with my values.

4. **Practicing Gratitude:**
Gratitude has become a daily practice that has significantly impacted my self-confidence and overall happiness. Taking a few moments each day to reflect on the things I'm grateful for, whether it's a supportive friend, a beautiful sunset, or a personal achievement, shifts my perspective towards positivity and abundance. This practice has nurtured a deep sense of gratitude within me and boosted my self-esteem.

5. **Surrounding Yourself with Supportive People:**
The power of positive and supportive relationships cannot be overstated. Surrounding myself with individuals who believe in

me, encourage me, and provide a safe space for growth has been instrumental in building my self-confidence. Their unwavering support and belief in my abilities have bolstered my confidence, helping me embrace challenges and pursue my dreams with greater determination.

6. **Embracing Personal Growth:**

Personal growth has been an ongoing journey for me, filled with exciting discoveries and occasional discomfort. By setting goals, challenging myself, and embracing new experiences, I've expanded my knowledge and capabilities. Stepping outside of my comfort zone has been both empowering and transformative, leading to increased self-confidence and a deeper belief in my own potential.

7. **Taking Care of Your Appearance:**

While true confidence goes beyond external appearances, taking care of how I present myself has positively influenced my self-image. Dressing in a way that makes me feel comfortable and confident, practicing good hygiene, and engaging in grooming habits that make me feel my best have all contributed to an enhanced sense of self-assurance. When we take pride in our appearance, it can positively impact our overall confidence.

8. **Celebrating Your Accomplishments:**

Celebrating my accomplishments, no matter how small, has been an essential part of my self-care and confidence-building journey. Acknowledging my hard work, giving myself credit for my achievements, and taking time to celebrate milestones has been incredibly empowering. It reinforces a positive self-image and encourages me to continue pushing forward and embracing new challenges.

By incorporating self-care practices and confidences boosters into our lives, we can nurture our well-being, cultivate a positive self-image, and lead a more fulfilling life. My own experiences have shown me that self-care and self-confidence are transformative forces that can enhance our overall happiness and resilience. Remember, this is a continuous journey, so be kind and patient with yourself as you embrace self-care and build your confidence, one step at a time.

Embracing Self-Acceptance and Confidence

In the realm of beauty, there is a profound connection between self-acceptance and confidence. When we embrace our true selves and exude confidence, we radiate a unique and captivating beauty. we will explore the transformative power of self-acceptance and how it intertwines with building unwavering confidence. By delving into practical strategies, we will unlock the secrets to embracing our beauty from within.

1. **Recognizing Your Inner Radiance:**
Beauty is not just about external appearances; it begins with recognizing the inner radiance that resides within each of us. Embrace your unique qualities, strengths, and inherent beauty. When you acknowledge and celebrate your authentic self, you unlock a captivating beauty that goes beyond what meets the eye.

2. **Nurturing Self-Love and Compassion:**

True beauty flourishes in an environment of self-love and compassion. Treat yourself with kindness, gentleness, and understanding. Embrace self-compassion by acknowledging that imperfections and mistakes are a natural part of being human. By cultivating self-love, you nourish a deep sense of acceptance and confidence that enhances your beauty.

3. **Letting Go of Unrealistic Standards:**

In a world obsessed with external perfection, it's vital to let go of unrealistic standards that hinder our self-acceptance. Embrace the beauty of diversity and celebrate your unique features. Release the pressure to conform and instead focus on highlighting your individuality. When you let go of societal expectations, you liberate yourself to fully embrace your authentic beauty.

4. **Embracing Self-Expression:**

Beauty is a form of self-expression that allows us to showcase our uniqueness and creativity. Embrace the power of self-expression through makeup, fashion, and personal style. Experiment with different looks and trends that resonate with your inner essence. Embracing self-expression empowers you to confidently express your beauty in ways that are true to yourself.

5. **Cultivating Inner Confidence:**

Confidence is the crowning jewel of beauty. Cultivating inner confidence begins with acknowledging your worth and embracing your strengths. Recognize your accomplishments, no matter how small, and celebrate them. Challenge self-doubt and negative self-talk by replacing them with positive affirmations. When you radiate inner confidence, your beauty becomes undeniable.

6. **Surrounding Yourself with Positive Influences:**

Surrounding yourself with positive influences is essential for cultivating self-acceptance and confidence. Seek out individuals who uplift and inspire you. Engage with communities that celebrate diversity and promote self-love. Surrounding yourself with positive influences creates a supportive environment that nurtures your beauty journey.

7. **Embracing Self-Care Rituals:**

Self-care rituals are a nurturing sanctuary that allows your beauty to flourish. Prioritize your well-being by engaging in skincare routines, haircare rituals, and overall wellness practices. Dedicate time to pamper yourself and indulge in activities that bring you joy and relaxation. When you prioritize self-care, you enhance your natural beauty from the inside out.

The path to embracing beauty begins with self-acceptance and confidence. By recognizing your inner radiance, nurturing self-love and compassion, letting go of unrealistic standards, embracing self-expression, cultivating inner confidence, surrounding yourself with positive influences, and indulging in self-care rituals, you unlock a beauty that is authentic and captivating. Embrace the journey, celebrate your uniqueness, and let your beauty shine brightly for the world to see.

Finding Joy in Everyday Life

Finding joy in everyday life is a transformative journey that stirs the depths of our being. It is an exploration of the soul, a quest to uncover the profound beauty that resides within the simplest moments. In the depths of our hearts, we yearn for happiness and fulfillment, and it is through embracing joy that we unlock the true essence of our existence. With every breath, we have the opportunity to infuse our lives with deep feelings of joy that transcend the ordinary and awaken our spirits.

Cultivating Gratitude:

Gratitude, oh how it opens the floodgates of profound emotion! It is a gentle whisper that echoes through our souls, reminding us of the abundance that surrounds us. As we cultivate gratitude, our hearts expand with appreciation for the blessings, both big and small, that grace our lives. It is in this deep feeling of gratitude that we discover the untamed joy that dances within us.

Embracing Mindfulness:

In the quietude of the present moment, there lies a treasure trove of deep feeling waiting to be unearthed. Through the practice of mindfulness, we immerse ourselves in the exquisite tapestry of sensations and experiences that unfold around us. Each breath becomes a conduit for heightened awareness, and within this awakened state, we find joy coursing through our veins, permeating every fiber of our being.

Pursuing Passions and Hobbies:

Passion, that fiery ember within us, beckons us to embrace the activities that ignite our souls. It is in the pursuit of our passions and hobbies that we discover a profound connection to our true selves. As we surrender to the ecstasy of creative expression or immerse ourselves in pursuits that bring us alive, a deep sense of joy envelops us, washing away the worries of the world.

Connecting with Loved Ones:
Ah, the profound beauty of human connection! It is in the loving embrace of our cherished ones that we discover a wellspring of deep feeling that transcends all boundaries. As we share laughter, tears, and intimate moments with those we hold dear, an indescribable joy arises within us, a symphony of love that resonates with the deepest chords of our hearts.

Seeking Beauty in the Everyday:
The world around us is a masterpiece, waiting to be witnessed with awe and reverence. Through open eyes and awakened senses, we discover beauty in the ordinary, in the dappled sunlight streaming through the leaves, in the gentle caress of a breeze, in the smiles exchanged between strangers. As we train our hearts to seek beauty in every nook and cranny of life, a profound sense of joy radiates from within, permeating our existence.

Practicing Acts of Kindness:
In the act of kindness, we tap into a wellspring of compassion that flows from the deepest recesses of our souls. As we extend a helping hand, offer a listening ear, or perform acts of selflessness, a deep feeling of joy envelops us. It is the exquisite joy that arises from knowing we have made a difference, no

matter how small, in someone else's life.

Embracing Playfulness and Laughter:
   Oh, the infectious melody of laughter! It is a balm for the soul, a symphony that reverberates through our being and reverberates into the world. As we embrace our inner child and surrender to moments of playfulness, joy bubbles up from within, untamed and uncontainable. In the uninhibited laughter that spills forth, we rediscover the pure, unadulterated joy of being alive.

Finding joy in everyday life is a journey that transcends the surface-level experiences and delves deep into the core of our being. Through cultivating gratitude, embracing mindfulness, pursuing passions, connecting with loved ones, seeking beauty, practicing acts of kindness, and embracing playfulness and laughter, we unlock the floodgates of deep feeling that reside within us. This journey, this exploration of joy, touches the very essence of our existence and transforms our lives from mundane to extraordinary. So, my dear souls, may you embark on this sacred path of joy and allow the deep well of feeling within you to overflow with the profound beauty that lies in every moment of your precious lives.

Prioritizing Self-Care in Your Routine

In the whirlwind of life's demands and responsibilities, it's easy to lose sight of our own well-being. However, prioritizing self-care is essential for maintaining a healthy body, mind, and spirit. In this section, we will explore practical ways to integrate self-care into your daily routine, ensuring that you nourish and rejuvenate yourself amidst life's busyness. By making self-care a non-negotiable priority, you will experience increased happiness, improved overall well-being, and a greater capacity to handle life's challenges.

1. Carving Out "Me Time":

Make it a habit to set aside dedicated time for yourself each day. This can be as simple as waking up 15 minutes earlier to enjoy a quiet cup of tea or taking a leisurely bath in the evening. Use this time to engage in activities that bring you joy, whether it's reading a book, practicing yoga, or indulging in a hobby. By deliberately creating space for yourself, you honor your needs and replenish your energy.

Example: Imagine starting your day with a peaceful morning ritual, sipping your favorite herbal tea while journaling or meditating. This quiet moment of self-reflection sets a positive tone for the rest of your day, allowing you to approach tasks with a calm and centered mindset.

2. Nurture Your Body with Movement:

Physical activity is not only beneficial for your physical health but also for your mental and emotional well-being. Find a form of exercise that you enjoy, whether it's dancing, jogging, practicing yoga, or taking long walks in nature. Engaging in regular exercise not only boosts your energy levels but also releases endorphins, the "feel-good" hormones that elevate your mood and reduce stress.

Example: Perhaps you incorporate a 30-minute dance session into your daily routine. Put on your favorite music and let yourself move freely, allowing the rhythm to awaken your body and uplift your spirits. Not only will you experience the physical benefits of exercise, but you will also feel a deep sense of joy and liberation as you dance to the beat of your own heart.

3. **Prioritize Restful Sleep:**
Quality sleep is a cornerstone of self-care. Establish a bedtime routine that promotes relaxation and ensures a restful night's sleep. Create a calming environment in your bedroom, free from distractions, and develop a soothing ritual before bed, such as reading a book, practicing deep breathing exercises, or listening to calming music. Aim for a consistent sleep schedule that allows you to wake up feeling refreshed and rejuvenated.

Example: Picture yourself winding down in the evening with a warm bath infused with lavender essential oil. As you soak in the soothing water, you let go of the day's stresses and prepare your body and mind for a peaceful slumber. This intentional act of self-care ensures that you awaken each morning feeling rested and ready to embrace the day.

4. **Nourish Your Body with Nutritious Foods:**
Fueling your body with nutritious foods is an act of self-love. Prioritize a balanced diet rich in fruits, vegetables, whole grains, and lean proteins. Incorporate foods that nourish not only your body but also your soul. Take the time to savor your meals, enjoying each bite mindfully and appreciating the flavors and textures.

Example: Consider preparing a vibrant and nourishing salad for lunch, filled with colorful vegetables, leafy greens, and a variety of textures and flavors. As you savor each bite, you are not only providing your body with essential nutrients but also taking a moment to honor your well-being and indulge in the simple pleasure of nourishing yourself from within.

5. **Practice Mindfulness and Stress-Reduction Techniques:**
Integrating mindfulness and stress-reduction techniques into your daily routine can significantly enhance your overall well-being. Engage in activities such as meditation, deep breathing exercises, or gentle yoga to cultivate a sense of inner calm and promote mental clarity. Set aside moments throughout the day to pause, breathe, and reconnect with the present moment.

Example: Imagine incorporating a brief mindfulness practice into your afternoon routine. Take a few minutes to sit in a quiet space, close your eyes, and focus on your breath. Allow yourself to fully immerse in the present moment, letting go of worries and distractions. This practice not only reduces stress but also cultivates a deep sense of inner peace and contentment.

Prioritizing self-care is not a luxury but a necessity for a fulfilling and balanced life. By carving out "me time," nurturing your body with movement and restful sleep, nourishing yourself with nutritious foods, and practicing mindfulness and stress-reduction techniques, you empower yourself to live with vitality, joy, and resilience. Embrace these practical examples of self-care and integrate them into your daily routine, knowing that by taking care of yourself, you are able to show up fully in all areas of your life.

7

Embracing the Wisdom and Beauty of Aging

Embracing the wisdom and beauty of aging is a profound journey of self-discovery and acceptance. As we grow older, we have the opportunity to cultivate a deep understanding of ourselves and the world around us. This section explores the ways in which we can embrace the wisdom and beauty that come with age, recognizing the transformative power of this natural process. By embracing our experiences, nurturing our inner selves, and celebrating the uniqueness of our individuality, we can fully embrace the journey of aging and radiate its inherent beauty.

1. **Honoring Life's Experiences:**

Aging grants us the gift of accumulated experiences. By acknowledging and honoring the lessons learned, the challenges overcome, and the growth achieved, we can embrace the wisdom that comes with a life well-lived. Each experience becomes a stepping stone on the path to self-discovery and personal development. By reflecting on our journey, we gain insight and perspective that allow us to navigate life's complexities with grace and understanding.

2. **Embracing Inner Beauty:**

As we age, true beauty transcends physical appearance. It is the inner radiance that emanates from a deep sense of self-acceptance, self-love, and compassion. Embracing inner beauty involves nurturing our inner selves through practices like self-care, self-reflection, and mindfulness. By cultivating gratitude for who we have become and celebrating our unique qualities, we can radiate a beauty that goes beyond age and societal expectations.

3. **Celebrating Individuality:**

Aging provides an opportunity to shed societal pressures and embrace our authentic selves. By celebrating our individuality, we allow our true essence to shine brightly. Embracing our passions, interests, and personal style empowers us to express ourselves freely and authentically. By embracing our uniqueness, we inspire others to do the same, creating a world where individuality is celebrated and cherished.

4. **Embracing Aging as a Journey:**

Aging is not a destination but a continuous journey of growth and transformation. Embracing this journey involves accepting the changes that come with age, whether they are physical, emotional, or spiritual. It means viewing aging as an opportunity for self-improvement, learning, and personal evolution. By embracing the unknown with curiosity and embracing each year as a new chapter, we can approach aging with a sense of excitement and anticipation.

Embracing the wisdom and beauty of aging is a deeply personal and transformative process. It requires self-reflection, self-acceptance, and an appreciation for the journey of life. By honoring our experiences, nurturing our inner selves, celebrating our individuality, and embracing aging as a continuous journey, we can embrace the beauty and wisdom that come with each passing year. As we radiate our inner light, we inspire others to do the same, creating a world where aging is celebrated as a remarkable and enriching part of life.

8

Conclusion

In conclusion, "Beauty Beyond 40" is a comprehensive guide that empowers women to embrace their beauty and confidently navigate the journey of aging. Throughout this exploration of beauty tips and practices for women aged 40 and beyond, we have delved into various aspects of self-care, skincare, makeup, haircare, fitness, wellness, and inner growth. The overarching message is that beauty knows no age limit and is a reflection of the inner strength, self-acceptance, and vitality that comes from embracing the fullness of life.

By understanding the changes that occur in mature skin, we can tailor our skincare routines to address specific concerns and maintain a healthy and radiant complexion. Incorporating anti-aging products and ingredients, such as serums and face oils, can further support the skin's resilience and youthful appearance. In the realm of makeup, we have explored tips and techniques for enhancing natural beauty, creating long-lasting looks, and embracing our unique features with confidence.

Furthermore, we have recognized the importance of haircare in maintaining healthy and vibrant locks, including strategies for dealing with thinning hair and hair loss. Whether it's through color and highlights or embracing the natural beauty of gray hair, we have learned that our hair is a canvas for self-expression and personal style.

Beyond the realm of physical beauty, we have delved into fitness and wellness practices that contribute to overall well-being. From stress reduction techniques to nutrition tips for healthy aging, we have emphasized the significance of self-care and self-preservation. By prioritizing our physical and mental well-being, we can enhance our vitality and radiate a sense of inner beauty that transcends age.

Equally important is the exploration of self-acceptance, self-confidence, and the embrace of change. Aging gracefully involves nurturing our inner selves, celebrating our unique qualities, and cultivating meaningful connections. By embracing self-acceptance and confidence, we can navigate the transitions and challenges that come with age with grace and resilience.

Ultimately, "Beauty Beyond 40" encourages women to embrace the journey of aging as an opportunity for self-discovery, personal growth, and the cultivation of wisdom. By prioritizing self-care, fostering inner beauty, and embracing our individuality, we can radiate a beauty that comes from a place of self-assuredness and authenticity. The tips and insights shared throughout this guide are meant to inspire and empower women

CONCLUSION

to celebrate their beauty and live their lives to the fullest.

As we conclude this exploration of beauty tips for women 40 and beyond, let us remember that true beauty knows no boundaries of age. It is a reflection of the inner light, confidence, and self-love that shines through at every stage of life. Let us embrace the beauty that comes with experience, wisdom, and self-acceptance, and inspire others to do the same. May every woman who embarks on this journey of beauty beyond 40 embrace her unique radiance and celebrate the remarkable beauty that lies within her.

```
I recommend you also read (TAURINE AND AGING THE
WONDER AMINO ACID)
```

Printed in Great Britain
by Amazon